TEMPORAL LOBE SEIZURES

TECHNIQUES FOR DEALING WITH TEMPORAL LOBE SEIZURES

DR. KATE .P

1

Contents

CHAPTER ONE

INTRODUCTION

The brain's temporal lobes, which are crucial for short-term memory and process emotions, are the source of temporal lobe seizures. These functions may be connected to certain symptoms of a temporal lobe seizure, such as strange emotions like exhilaration, deja vu, or dread.

Even during a seizure involving the temporal lobe, consciousness may persist. In more severe seizures, you may appear awake but not responding. You might make repetitive, meaningless gestures with your lips and hands.

The reason of temporal lobe seizures is frequently unclear, but it could be caused by a scar or anatomical defect in the temporal lobe. Medicine is used to treat seizures caused by the temporal lobe. Surgery might be an option for some people whose condition doesn't improve with medicine.

Symptoms

A temporal lobe seizure may be preceded by an atypical feeling (aura), which serves as a warning. Not everyone with auras remembers them, and not everyone with temporal lobe seizures experiences auras.

In actuality, the aura is just a straightforward partial or focal seizure that doesn't affect consciousness. Aura examples include:

An unexpected feeling of unwarranted fear

A sensation of déjà vu, or the idea that something has happened before

An abrupt or peculiar taste or smell

An abdominal rising feeling

Partial complex or focal dyscognitive seizures are a type of temporal lobe seizures that can occasionally make it difficult to react to other people. The typical duration of this kind of temporal lobe seizure is between 30 and 2 minutes. Typical indications and manifestations include of:

loss of awareness of one's environment

gazing

Smacking your lips

recurrent chewing or swallowing

strange finger actions, like plucking motions

Following a seizure of the temporal lobe, you might have:

a phase of disorientation and trouble speaking

not being able to remember what happened during the seizure

Not realizing one had experienced a seizure

excessive drowsiness

Seizures that begin as temporal lobe seizures can progress to generalized tonic-clonic seizures, often known as grand mal seizures, which are characterized by convulsions and unconsciousness.

When to visit a physician

Seek medical guidance in the following situations:

If you believe that you or your kid is experiencing seizures

When seizures become more frequent or severe and there's no apparent reason for it

When fresh seizure indicators or symptoms surface

Seek immediate medical attention if:

More than five minutes pass during a seizure.

After the seizure ends, the person doesn't recover fully or as soon as usual.

Repeated seizures occur during a single day.

Reasons

The etiology of temporal lobe seizures is frequently yet unclear. However, several factors, such as the following, may contribute to them:

traumatic brain damage

Meningitis or encephalitis infections, or a history of such diseases a procedure that results in gliosis, or scarring, in the hippocampal region of the temporal lobe

brain blood vessel abnormalities

a stroke

brain growths

genetic disorders

Different electrical activity is produced by brain cells during regular waking and sleeping. A convulsion or seizure may happen if numerous brain cells' electrical activity synchronizes improperly.

A focal seizure occurs if this occurs in a single location of the brain. A partial seizure that starts in one of the temporal lobes is known as a temporal lobe seizure.

COMMITMENTS

Recurrent seizures in the temporal lobe can eventually lead to shrinkage of the hippocampal region of the brain, which is involved in learning and memory. Decreases in brain cells in this region may lead to memory issues.

Getting Ready for Your Consultation

After visiting your family physician or general practitioner, you will probably be sent to a physician who specializes in problems of the neurological system (a neurologist).

The following details will help you get ready for your appointment.

What you're capable of

Note all of the symptoms that you or your kid have experienced, even if they don't seem to be connected to seizures. Take note of the different seizure types. Do some, for instance, have a greater effect on the left side of the body than the right, or vice versa? Some have an impact on speech, whereas others don't?

Enumerate all of the vitamins, minerals, and prescription drugs that you, or your child, are taking, along with their dosages. Note the reasons you stopped taking them, including any negative effects or ineffectiveness.

CHAPTER TWO

To assist you recall the information you are given at your appointment, ask a family member to go with you. Furthermore, someone watching the seizures might be able to describe them more accurately than you can because seizures can cause memory loss.

If at all feasible, have a friend or family member use a cellphone or other video recorder to capture the seizure on camera.

Prepare a list of inquiries for your physician

You may maximize your time with your doctor by preparing a list of questions in advance. Some inquiries to make regarding temporal lobe seizures are as follows:

Is epilepsy the diagnosis?

Will there be additional seizures? Will there be a variety of seizures?

Which tests are required? Do you need to prepare differently for these tests?

Which of the available treatments would you suggest?

What kinds of adverse effects might a treatment cause?

Is it possible to have surgery?

Do I need to limit my activities? What concerns do I have with safety?

Is this illness perhaps fatal? How can I reduce the dangers that come with having my condition?

Is there a generic version of the medication you are recommending?

Are there any pamphlets or other printed things that I could take? Which websites would you suggest?

Please feel free to ask any more questions.

What to anticipate from your physician

You should expect to be asked a lot of questions by your doctor, including:

When did your child or you start experiencing symptoms?

Before the convulsions, were there any strange sensations you noticed?

What is the frequency of seizures?

What constitutes a normal seizure?

What is the duration of the seizures?

Do the seizures happen in groups?

Do they all have the same appearance, or have you or others observed distinct seizure behaviors?

During a seizure, does the head or body of you or your child turn in one direction?

Does speech change in the early stages of a seizure?

Has a seizure caused any injuries to you or your child?

Following the seizure, how would you characterize yourself or your child?

Which drugs have you and your kid tried? Which dosages were applied?

Have you ever attempted mixing medications?

Do conditions like illness or lack of sleep seem to be triggers for seizures?

assessments and diagnosis

Health background

The majority of patients who experience temporal lobe seizures are not aware of the seizures, thus your doctor will require a thorough account of the seizures, preferably from a spectator.

neurological assessment

It is likely that your doctor will do a neurological exam if you or your kid has experienced a seizure that includes testing:

Backwards

tone of the muscles

strength of muscles

sensory ability

Walk

Positioning

Harmony

Fairness

To evaluate your reasoning, discernment, and recollection, he or she might also pose questions.

Scanners and blood tests

If there are any concerns that might be causing or initiating the seizures, blood tests might be prescribed.

Tests or scans intended to identify anomalies in the brain can also be recommended by your physician.

the electroencephalogram (EEG). Your scalp-attached electrodes capture your brain's electrical activity, which is displayed on an EEG. Individuals who do not experience seizures frequently exhibit alterations in their brain wave patterns. Occasionally, the EEG can provide information on the kind of seizures you're experiencing.

Under some circumstances, your physician might suggest hospitalized video-EEG monitoring. This enables your physician to precisely match your EEG pattern to the actions seen during a seizure, second by second. In order to choose the best course of action and confirm that the diagnosis of seizures is accurate, this can assist your doctor in precisely diagnosing the kind of seizure problem you are experiencing.

magnetic resonance imaging (MRI). Your brain is shown in great detail on an MRI machine. An MRI's anomalies can reveal information about the underlying cause of seizures, even though many patients with epilepsy and seizures have normal tests.

A padded table that slips into the MRI machine will be used for your test positioning. In order to enhance accuracy, a brace will immobilize your head. The MRI test is painless, but the small space within the machine causes claustrophobia in certain people. Please let your doctor know before the study if you suspect you could experience this reaction.

PCT stands for single-photon emission tomography. One scan during a seizure and one during a nonseizure period, conducted on different days, are needed for SPECT imaging, which is sometimes employed when the location of seizure initiation is unknown. An injection of radioactive material is made at each scan.

To determine which part of the brain was most active during the seizure, the scans are compared. Next, the final picture is placed on top of the MRI. In order to assist the surgeons, this is used in conjunction with EEG data.

Pharmaceuticals and supplements

Medications

Treating temporal lobe seizures involves a variety of drugs. Medication alone, however, is not always effective in controlling seizures, and side effects such as weariness, weight gain, and dizziness are frequent.

When determining the best course of therapy, talk to your doctor about any potential adverse effects. Furthermore enquire about potential interactions between the medications you take for seizures and other conditions, such as oral contraceptives.

Procedure

Consideration for surgery may be given if the seizures from your temporal lobe are unresponsive to medicine. Surgery does away with or significantly lessens seizures in certain individuals.

Seizures surgery does, however, include some dangers, like any operation. Neurological issues may arise, and it could not be successful. With your surgeon and neurologist, go over the potential hazards.

The following situations usually rule out surgery:

Vital brain activities are carried out by the area of the brain causing your seizures.

Multiple locations are the source of your seizures.

It is not possible to identify your seizure focus.

Getting ready for surgical procedures

Discuss the procedure you're thinking about having done with your surgeon regarding their experience, success and complication rates. Also, before having surgery, you might wish to get a second opinion.

An extensive assessment

cerebral MRI scans

employing video records and EEG to track your seizures at a hospital-based monitoring unit

subsequent to surgery

In order to help prevent seizures, most people must continue taking their medications. Medication can be cut back on and even stopped sometimes if surgery seems to be beneficial.

Vagus nerve stimulation

CHAPTER THREE

In the event that drugs are ineffectual or have severe adverse effects, a vagus nerve stimulator may be a possibility. Your collarbone is exposed when the stimulator is inserted in your chest. Your neck's vagus nerve receives wires from the stimulator.

By using a magnet to trigger it, users can set the device to turn on and off at specific times. Seizures are not detected by this apparatus. Even though it's typically well tolerated, medication should not be substituted with it.

Cyber stimulation that reacts

A device that treats seizures that don't respond to medication has received FDA approval. When the apparatus notices seizure activity, it stimulates the affected area electrically. Connected to a battery-operated generator implanted in the skull near the brain, the device is inserted either on the surface of the brain or inside the brain tissue.

Extended brain activation

Placing electrodes into the thalamus, a region of the brain, is known as deep brain stimulation. For the treatment of seizures, this therapy is not currently FDA-approved. Treating seizures that are unresponsive to medicine may benefit from it in certain, carefully chosen circumstances. Additional research is required.

Seizure and pregnancy

Pregnancy should always be planned, that much is certain. Typically, healthy pregnancies can occur in women using medication for seizures. Yet, it is well recognized that taking some drugs while pregnant increases the chance of birth abnormalities. One such prescription is valproic acid (Depakene).

It is generally advised against stopping medication during pregnancy due to the danger of seizures to the growing fetus. Take your doctor through these dangers. Preconception counseling is crucial for women who have seizures because pregnancy might change a person's medication dosage.

Proprietary folic acid, taken daily prior to conception, can help prevent birth abnormalities associated with seizure medicine if you are taking it and may get pregnant.

Multiple drug-using mothers are thought to be at an increased risk of birth abnormalities. With other medications, if your seizures are not adequately controlled, talk to your doctor about the possible hazards.

Anti-seizure drugs and birth control

Oral contraceptive (birth control) pill may become less effective when taken with some anti-seizure drugs. Ask your doctor if there are any drug interactions with your oral contraceptive and whether you should look into other methods of birth control if getting pregnant is a top priority.

Domestic medicine and lifestyle

If you experience a seizure while engaging in certain activities, it could be dangerous. Some of the activities are:

Diving. Make careful you wear a life preserver and avoid going into the water alone.

taking a shower. The risk of drowning increases when taking a bath. instead take a shower.

operating at a height. Seizures can cause falls.

operating machinery, like as an automobile. For those with a history of seizures, there are license limits that apply in every state. Every state has its own set of rules.

To assist first responders, think about donning a medical alert bracelet. Along with your medicine allergies, the information on who to call in an emergency should be listed on the wristband.

Adapting and offering support

Seizures can have an impact on your life even if they are managed. Because people might not recognize the strange behavior as a seizure, temporal lobe seizures may provide even greater challenges to coping. Living with the continual fear of another seizure can irritate both children and adults. Children may be bullied or embarrassed by their illness.

Speaking with people going through similar experiences could be beneficial. They may provide guidance or coping mechanisms you haven't considered in addition to their assistance.

For teens and adults who experience seizures as well as parents of children who experience seizures, the Epilepsy Foundation offers a network of support groups and online forums.

THE END

www.ingramcontent.com/pod-product-compliance
Lightning Source LLC
Chambersburg PA
CBHW070937290526
45795CB00003B/1053